CONTENTS

INTRODUCTION

In a world marked by ever-changing health trends and quick-fix solutions, it's often challenging to discern the path to genuine well-being. Amidst this sea of information, there emerges a beacon of science-backed wisdom that stands as a testament to the power of balanced nutrition and holistic health the Dietary Approaches to Stop Hypertension, or the DASH diet.

Imagine a journey that doesn't promise overnight transformations or drastic measures, but instead offers a transformative approach to nourishing your body, mind, and soul. This journey is precisely what the DASH diet represents a voyage towards embracing health, vitality, and a brighter future.

As we delve into the pages of this book, we embark on a remarkable expedition—one that will unravel the intricacies of the DASH diet and guide us towards a more profound understanding of its principles, benefits, and the science that underpins its success. Together, we will journey through the world of nutrient-rich foods, explore the art of mindful eating, and discover the profound impact that our dietary choices can have on our overall well-being.

Beyond the realm of mere food, the DASH diet introduces us to a holistic approach to health—one that considers not only the nutritional value of what we consume, but also the importance of physical activity, stress management, sleep, and a positive mindset. It is a lifestyle that resonates with the rhythm of life itself, emphasizing the harmonious interplay of various elements that contribute to our vitality.

As we embark on this expedition, we invite you to open your mind, heart, and palate to the possibilities that the DASH diet offers. Whether you're seeking to manage your blood pressure, enhance your cardiovascular health, maintain a healthy weight, or simply cultivate a more vibrant existence, the principles of the DASH diet are here to guide you.

This book serves as your compass, guiding you through the intricate landscapes of nutrition, offering practical tips for grocery shopping, meal planning, and dining out, and addressing common misconceptions that may obscure your path. With each chapter, you'll gain a deeper appreciation for the remarkable synergy between the foods we eat and the life we lead.

As you turn these pages, remember that you are not alone on this journey. Together, we will unravel the mysteries of the DASH diet, embracing its principles, and navigating the seas of health and wellness with wisdom, determination, and joy. So, let us embark on this adventure—an adventure that promises not only a healthier tomorrow but a richer, more fulfilling today.

CHAPTER ONE

Introduction to the DASH Diet

Understanding DASH: Dietary Approaches to Stop Hypertension

The Dietary Approaches to Stop Hypertension (DASH) is not just another fad diet; it's a scientifically designed eating plan that aims to combat hypertension, commonly known as high blood pressure. This comprehensive dietary strategy was developed by the National Heart, Lung, and Blood Institute (NHLBI) to address the growing concern of hypertension and its associated health risks. DASH stands out from other diets due to its focus on a balanced, nutrient-rich approach rather than strict calorie restrictions.

At its core, the DASH diet emphasizes the consumption of whole foods, such as fruits, vegetables, whole grains, lean proteins, and low-fat dairy products. It places particular emphasis on reducing sodium intake, which is a major contributor to elevated blood pressure. This is achieved by minimizing the consumption of high-sodium processed foods, such as canned soups, salty snacks, and fast food, which are all too prevalent in modern diets.

A key aspect of DASH is its attention to nutrient density. Rather than merely counting calories, DASH encourages individuals to prioritize foods that are rich in essential vitamins, minerals, and dietary fiber. By doing so, the diet not only helps manage blood pressure but also contributes to overall well-being. The abundance of potassium, magnesium, and calcium-rich foods in the DASH diet has been linked to improved cardiovascular health and reduced risk of chronic diseases.

The Science Behind DASH: How It Promotes Health

The scientific principles underlying the DASH diet are rooted in decades of research. Clinical studies have consistently demonstrated its effectiveness in reducing blood pressure and enhancing cardiovascular health. The diet's emphasis on consuming potassium-rich foods like bananas, spinach, and beans plays a pivotal role in blood pressure regulation. Potassium helps counteract the effects of sodium by promoting relaxation of blood vessel walls, leading to improved blood flow and reduced pressure on arterial walls.

Furthermore, the DASH diet promotes the consumption of dietary fiber, which offers a range of health benefits. Fiber-rich foods, including whole grains, fruits, and vegetables, contribute to sustained feelings of fullness and assist in weight management. Moreover, dietary fiber supports digestive health, helps stabilize blood sugar levels, and even aids in lowering cholesterol levels.

The inclusion of lean protein sources, such as poultry, fish, and legumes, in the DASH diet contributes to the maintenance and repair of body tissues. These proteins are lower in saturated fat compared to red meat, aligning with the diet's heart-healthy objectives. The diet also encourages the intake of healthy fats, primarily derived from sources like nuts, seeds, and olive oil, which have been associated with reduced inflammation and improved cardiovascular function.

Benefits of DASH Beyond Blood Pressure Management

While the primary focus of the DASH diet is to manage and prevent hypertension, its benefits extend far beyond blood pressure regulation. By promoting a balanced and nutrient-rich eating pattern, the DASH diet contributes to overall health and well-being in various ways.

- Weight Management: The DASH diet's emphasis on whole foods and portion control naturally supports weight management. Its high-fiber content helps individuals feel fuller for longer, reducing the likelihood of overeating. Unlike many fad diets that rely on drastic calorie restrictions, the DASH diet offers a sustainable approach to weight loss and maintenance.
- Diabetes Prevention and Management: The DASH diet's emphasis on whole grains, lean proteins, and low-fat dairy products can help regulate blood sugar levels, making it beneficial for individuals with diabetes or those at risk of developing the condition. The diet's focus on complex carbohydrates and nutrient-dense foods helps prevent rapid spikes in blood sugar.
- Heart Health: Beyond blood pressure reduction, the DASH diet significantly improves overall cardiovascular health. Its emphasis on heart-healthy fats, such as monounsaturated fats found in olive oil and avocados, contributes to lowering the risk of heart disease by reducing inflammation and improving cholesterol levels.

- Cancer Prevention: The abundance of fruits and vegetables in the DASH diet provides a rich source of antioxidants and phytochemicals, which are known to play a role in cancer prevention. These compounds help protect cells from damage and promote overall cellular health.
- Bone Health: The DASH diet's inclusion of dairy products and other calcium-rich foods supports bone health, reducing the risk of osteoporosis and fractures. Additionally, the diet's emphasis on magnesium-rich foods further contributes to bone density and overall skeletal well-being.
- Long-Term Sustainability: One of the most remarkable aspects of the DASH diet is its long-term sustainability. Unlike many trendy diets that are difficult to maintain over time, the DASH diet provides a balanced and flexible approach to eating that can be adopted for life. This makes it more likely for individuals to stick with the diet and reap its health benefits in the long run.

In conclusion, the Dietary Approaches to Stop Hypertension (DASH) diet represents a scientifically backed approach to promoting health and well-being. With its emphasis on whole foods, nutrient density, and balanced eating, DASH not only effectively manages blood pressure but also offers a range of additional health benefits. From weight management and diabetes prevention to heart health and cancer protection, the DASH diet's holistic approach contributes to a healthier and more vibrant life. As individuals adopt the principles of DASH and make them a part of their daily dietary habits, they pave the way for a future marked by improved overall health and reduced risk of chronic diseases

Foundations of the DASH Diet
Key Principles and Guidelines of the DASH Diet

The DASH diet is grounded in a set of key principles and guidelines that provide a roadmap for adopting a healthier eating pattern and effectively managing blood pressure. These principles, backed by scientific research, guide individuals toward making informed dietary choices that promote overall well-being. Let's delve into some of the fundamental principles that form the foundation of the DASH diet:

- Rich in Fruits and Vegetables: The DASH diet places a strong emphasis on consuming a variety of fruits and vegetables. These nutrient-dense foods provide essential vitamins, minerals, and dietary fiber that contribute to optimal health. They also deliver antioxidants that help protect cells from damage and reduce inflammation.
- Whole Grains: The diet encourages the consumption of whole grains over refined grains. Whole grains, such as brown rice, quinoa, and whole wheat, are packed with fiber and nutrients that support digestive health, provide sustained energy, and contribute to a feeling of fullness.
- Lean Protein Sources: The DASH diet emphasizes lean protein sources, such as poultry, fish, beans, and legumes. These protein-rich foods are lower in saturated fat, which supports heart health, and they provide essential amino acids for tissue repair and growth.
- Low-Fat Dairy: The diet recommends low-fat or fat-free dairy products, such as yogurt and milk.

These dairy options supply calcium and vitamin D, crucial for bone health, without the added saturated fat content found in full-fat dairy.

- Nuts, Seeds, and Healthy Fats: Incorporating nuts, seeds, and healthy fats like olive oil and avocado contributes to a balanced intake of monounsaturated and polyunsaturated fats. These fats have been associated with heart health and reduced inflammation.
- Reduced Sodium Intake: A cornerstone of the DASH diet is reducing sodium consumption. Cutting back on high-sodium processed foods and using herbs, spices, and other flavor enhancers can help manage blood pressure by minimizing water retention and stress on blood vessel walls.
- Moderation of Sweets and Added Sugars: While not entirely eliminating sweets, the DASH diet promotes moderation in the consumption of added sugars. This guideline aligns with the overall goal of promoting a nutrient-rich diet while minimizing empty calories.
- Balanced and Varied Diet: The DASH diet encourages a well-rounded and diverse eating pattern. By incorporating a wide range of foods, individuals can ensure they're getting a comprehensive array of nutrients to support overall health.

Food Groups Emphasized in the DASH Diet

The DASH diet focuses on a selection of food groups that work in harmony to create a balanced and health-promoting eating pattern. Each food group contributes unique nutrients that collectively support cardiovascular health, blood pressure management, and overall well-being. Here's a breakdown of the food groups emphasized in the DASH diet:

- Fruits and Vegetables: These form the cornerstone of the DASH diet. Rich in vitamins, minerals, and antioxidants, fruits and vegetables provide essential nutrients that help regulate blood pressure, support immune function, and reduce the risk of chronic diseases.
- Whole Grains: Whole grains are integral to the DASH diet's fiber content. They stabilize blood sugar levels, contribute to satiety, and promote digestive health. Incorporating whole grains like whole wheat, oats, and barley adds a nutritious foundation to meals.
- Lean Proteins: Lean protein sources, such as poultry, fish, beans, and legumes, are excellent alternatives to red meat. They provide essential amino acids without the saturated fat content that can contribute to heart disease.
- Low-Fat Dairy: Low-fat or fat-free dairy options supply calcium, vitamin D, and protein without the excess saturated fat found in full-fat dairy products. Yogurt, milk, and cheese from these sources contribute to bone health and overall nutrition.
- Nuts, Seeds, and Healthy Fats: Nuts, seeds, and healthy fats like olive oil are rich in heart-healthy monounsaturated and polyunsaturated fats. These fats support cardiovascular health, reduce inflammation, and provide a source of sustained energy.

Portion Control and Caloric Considerations

While the DASH diet does not emphasize strict calorie counting, portion control plays a vital role in its effectiveness. Monitoring portion sizes helps individuals manage their caloric intake and achieve their health and weight goals. Here are some practical considerations related to portion control and caloric intake within the DASH diet:

- Balanced Meals: Aim to create well-balanced meals that include a variety of food groups. Fill half of your plate with fruits and vegetables, one-quarter with lean protein, and one-quarter with whole grains.
- Mindful Eating: Practice mindful eating by paying attention to hunger and fullness cues. Eat slowly, savor each bite, and stop when you feel comfortably satisfied, not overly full.
- Nutrient-Dense Choices: Prioritize nutrient-dense foods that provide essential vitamins, minerals, and fiber without excessive calories. These foods contribute to a feeling of fullness and support overall health.
- Healthy Snacking: Choose healthy snacks, such as a handful of nuts, fresh fruit, or vegetable sticks with hummus. These options help curb hunger between meals and prevent overeating during main meals.
- Hydration: Drink plenty of water throughout the day. Sometimes, thirst can be mistaken for hunger, leading to unnecessary snacking.
- Sodium Awareness: Be cautious of hidden sources of sodium, especially in processed foods. Excess

sodium can lead to water retention and increased blood pressure.

- Customization: The DASH diet can be tailored to individual calorie needs. Those aiming for weight loss may need to adjust portion sizes slightly to create a calorie deficit, while those aiming for weight maintenance should focus on balance and moderation.

In summary, the DASH diet's key principles and guidelines emphasize a balanced and nutrient-rich eating pattern that supports blood pressure management and overall health. By prioritizing whole foods, portion control, and mindful eating, individuals can harness the power of the DASH diet to achieve their health goals and enjoy a more vibrant and energized lifestyle.

The DASH Diet Food Groups
Incorporating Fruits and Vegetables for Nutrient-Rich Meals

Fruits and vegetables are the vibrant heart of the DASH diet, providing an array of essential nutrients that contribute to overall health and well-being. These colorful, nutrient-dense foods are brimming with vitamins, minerals, antioxidants, and dietary fiber that play a pivotal role in maintaining a healthy body and managing blood pressure.

Incorporating fruits and vegetables into your meals doesn't have to be a monotonous task. Instead, it offers an exciting opportunity to explore diverse flavors and textures. Start your day with a burst of vitality by adding fresh berries, sliced bananas, or diced mango to your breakfast cereal or yogurt. For lunch, consider creating a vibrant salad with mixed greens, cherry tomatoes, cucumber slices, and a variety of colorful bell peppers. Incorporate vegetables into your main dishes by adding sautéed spinach, broccoli, or zucchini to pasta or stir-fries.

To maximize the nutritional benefits of fruits and vegetables, aim for a variety of colors. Each hue signifies a unique set of nutrients and antioxidants. Dark leafy greens like kale and spinach provide an excellent source of vitamin K and folate, while orange vegetables like carrots and sweet potatoes are rich in beta-carotene, a precursor to vitamin A. Including a rainbow of produce in your meals not only enhances visual appeal but also ensures a well-rounded intake of vitamins, minerals, and phytochemicals that contribute to your overall health.

Grains and Their Whole Grain Varieties in a Balanced Diet

Whole grains are a cornerstone of the DASH diet, delivering a steady supply of complex carbohydrates, fiber, and essential nutrients. Unlike refined grains, which have been stripped of their bran and germ layers, whole grains retain their full nutritional value and provide a host of health benefits. By incorporating whole grain varieties into your diet, you can support heart health, regulate blood sugar levels, and promote digestive wellness.

Whole grains come in a diverse array of options, each with its own unique flavor and texture. Brown rice, quinoa, whole wheat, barley, and oats are just a few examples of whole grains that can easily be integrated into your meals. Opt for whole grain bread, pasta, and cereal to ensure you're getting the full nutritional package.

To create balanced and nutrient-rich meals, use whole

grains as a base for dishes. For example, build a satisfying bowl with cooked quinoa or brown rice topped with lean protein, vegetables, and a drizzle of olive oil. Incorporate whole grain pasta into your favorite pasta dishes, and experiment with different types of whole grain bread for sandwiches and toast.

Lean Proteins: Lean Meat, Poultry, Fish, Nuts, and Legumes

Lean proteins are essential components of the DASH diet, providing a source of amino acids necessary for tissue repair, growth, and overall health. These proteins offer a valuable alternative to red meat, which is often higher in saturated fat and can contribute to heart disease. By incorporating lean protein sources, you can support cardiovascular health, manage blood pressure, and maintain muscle mass.

Lean meats, such as skinless poultry and trimmed cuts of pork or beef, offer a protein-packed foundation for meals. Opt for baking, grilling, or broiling these meats to minimize added fats. Fish, particularly fatty fish like salmon, mackerel, and trout, provide omega-3 fatty acids that have been linked to heart health and reduced inflammation.

Plant-based sources of protein, such as nuts and legumes, offer an excellent alternative for individuals looking to reduce their meat consumption. Nuts, including almonds, walnuts, and pistachios, provide healthy fats and protein. Incorporate them into your diet by adding them to salads, oatmeal, or yogurt. Legumes, which include beans, lentils, and chickpeas, are rich in fiber and protein. Use them to create hearty soups, stews, and meatless chili.

Dairy Delights: Low-Fat Dairy and Dairy Alternatives

Dairy products and dairy alternatives are essential components of the DASH diet, providing valuable sources of calcium, vitamin D, and protein. These nutrients are crucial for maintaining bone health, supporting immune function, and promoting overall well-being. The DASH diet encourages the consumption of low-fat or fat-free dairy products to reduce saturated fat intake while reaping the benefits of dairy.

Low-fat yogurt, milk, and cheese are versatile dairy options that can be incorporated into a variety of dishes. Enjoy a serving of yogurt topped with fresh fruit and a sprinkle of nuts for a nutritious breakfast or snack. Use low-fat milk as a base for smoothies or to create creamy sauces for pasta dishes.

For those who prefer dairy alternatives, fortified plant-based options like almond milk, soy milk, and oat milk provide an adequate source of calcium and vitamin D. Be sure to choose unsweetened varieties to minimize added sugars. These dairy alternatives can be used in the same way as traditional dairy products, such as in cereals, coffee, and baking.

Incorporating these dairy delights into your meals not only supports bone health but also contributes to the overall nutrient density of your diet. Whether you choose low-fat dairy or dairy alternatives, these options play a valuable role in creating a balanced and health-promoting eating pattern as outlined by the DASH diet.

Crafting a DASH Diet Meal Plan

Building Breakfast: Delicious and Nutrient-Packed Options

Starting your day with a nutrient-packed breakfast sets the tone for healthy eating and energy throughout the day. The DASH diet offers a variety of delicious options that combine essential food groups to create balanced and satisfying breakfasts.

Option 1: Greek Yogurt Parfait

- Layer low-fat Greek yogurt with mixed berries, a drizzle of honey, and a sprinkle of chopped nuts. This parfait provides protein, probiotics, antioxidants, and healthy fats to fuel your morning.

Option 2: Veggie Omelette

- Whisk together egg whites with chopped spinach, tomatoes, and bell peppers. Cook in a non-stick pan and top with a sprinkle of low-fat cheese. Serve with whole grain toast for added fiber.

Option 3: Overnight Oats

- Combine rolled oats with low-fat milk or a dairy alternative, chia seeds, and your favorite fruits. Let it sit in the refrigerator overnight for a convenient and filling breakfast.

Lunchtime Creations: Salads, Sandwiches, and More

Lunch is an opportunity to incorporate a variety of nutrient-dense foods into your day. Create satisfying meals that include lean proteins, whole grains, and plenty of vegetables.

Option 1: Grilled Chicken Salad

- Combine grilled chicken breast, mixed greens, cherry tomatoes, cucumbers, and a sprinkle of feta cheese. Top with a light vinaigrette made with olive oil and balsamic vinegar.

Option 2: Turkey and Avocado Wrap

- Fill a whole grain wrap with sliced turkey, avocado, spinach, and shredded carrots. Add a dollop of hummus for extra flavor and creaminess.

Option 3: Lentil and Vegetable Soup

- Prepare a hearty lentil and vegetable soup with carrots, celery, onion, and spinach. Serve with a side of whole grain bread for a comforting and nourishing lunch.

Wholesome Dinners: Recipes for Flavorful DASH-Compliant Meals

Dinner is an opportunity to gather with loved ones and enjoy a satisfying meal. Prepare DASH-compliant dinners that prioritize lean proteins, whole grains, and a colorful array of vegetables.

Option 1: Baked Salmon with Quinoa and Roasted Vegetables

- Season salmon fillets with herbs and bake until flaky. Serve over cooked quinoa and a side of roasted broccoli, bell peppers, and zucchini.

Option 2: Stir-Fried Tofu and Vegetables

- Stir-fry tofu with a medley of colorful vegetables, such as bell peppers, snap peas, and broccoli. Use a light soy sauce-based sauce and serve over brown rice.

Option 3: Mediterranean Chickpea Salad

- Combine chickpeas, diced cucumbers, cherry tomatoes, red onion, and Kalamata olives. Toss with a lemon-oregano vinaigrette and crumbled feta cheese for a refreshing and flavorful salad.

Smart Snacking: Navigating Between-Meal Munchies

Smart snacking is an integral part of the DASH diet, helping to stabilize blood sugar levels and prevent overeating during main meals. Choose nutrient-rich options that provide sustained energy and satiety.

Option 1: Hummus and Veggie Sticks

- Dip carrot, celery, and bell pepper sticks into a serving of hummus. This combination offers a satisfying crunch along with fiber and protein.

Option 2: Mixed Nuts and Berries

- Create a small trail mix with a handful of mixed nuts and dried berries. The combination of healthy fats and antioxidants makes for a satisfying snack.

Option 3: Greek Yogurt and Fruit

- Enjoy a serving of low-fat Greek yogurt topped with fresh berries and a drizzle of honey. The protein and probiotics in yogurt promote fullness and digestive health.

Incorporating these breakfast, lunch, dinner, and snack options into your daily routine can help you adhere to the principles of the DASH diet while enjoying a variety of delicious and nutrient-rich meals. By prioritizing whole foods, lean proteins, and a colorful array of fruits and vegetables, you can support your overall health and well-being while effectively managing your blood pressure.

CHAPTER TWO

Managing Hypertension: How the DASH Diet Lowers Blood Pressure

One of the primary goals of the DASH diet is to manage and prevent hypertension, or high blood pressure. The diet's effectiveness in lowering blood pressure is rooted in its emphasis on specific nutrients and food groups that have been shown to have a positive impact on cardiovascular health.

- Sodium Reduction: The DASH diet's emphasis on reducing sodium intake is a critical factor in blood pressure management. High sodium intake can lead to fluid retention and increased pressure on blood vessel walls. By minimizing processed foods and incorporating fresh, whole foods, the DASH diet helps lower sodium consumption, thus reducing the risk of elevated blood pressure.
- Potassium-Rich Foods: The DASH diet encourages the consumption of potassium-rich foods, such as fruits, vegetables, and legumes. Potassium helps regulate fluid balance and supports the relaxation of blood vessel walls, contributing to improved blood flow and lower blood pressure.
- Calcium and Magnesium: The diet's focus on low-

fat dairy products and whole grains provides essential minerals like calcium and magnesium. These minerals are associated with improved blood vessel function and contribute to blood pressure regulation.

- Fiber and Antioxidants: The abundance of fiber and antioxidants from fruits, vegetables, and whole grains in the DASH diet supports overall cardiovascular health. Fiber helps maintain blood sugar levels and supports weight management, both of which contribute to blood pressure control.

Weight Management: Using DASH for Sustainable Weight Loss

The DASH diet isn't just about managing blood pressure; it also offers a sensible approach to weight management and sustainable weight loss. By prioritizing nutrient-dense foods and portion control, the DASH diet provides a framework for achieving and maintaining a healthy weight.

- Satiety and Fullness: The high fiber content of the DASH diet helps individuals feel fuller for longer periods, reducing the likelihood of overeating and promoting a sense of satiety.
- Balanced Nutrient Intake: The DASH diet's emphasis on a balanced intake of protein, carbohydrates, and fats ensures that your body receives the nutrients it needs for optimal functioning, which can lead to more effective weight management.
- Mindful Eating: The DASH diet encourages

mindful eating practices, such as paying attention to hunger and fullness cues. This approach helps prevent overconsumption and promotes a healthier relationship with food.

- Long-Term Sustainability: Unlike many restrictive diets, the DASH diet offers a sustainable approach to weight management. By promoting a variety of nutrient-rich foods and avoiding drastic calorie restrictions, individuals are more likely to adhere to the diet over the long term.

Diabetes and DASH: Controlling Blood Sugar Levels

The principles of the DASH diet align well with the dietary recommendations for individuals with diabetes or those at risk of developing the condition. The diet's emphasis on whole foods, complex carbohydrates, and controlled portions can contribute to better blood sugar control.

- Steady Blood Sugar: The DASH diet's focus on whole grains and fiber-rich foods helps regulate blood sugar levels and prevents rapid spikes and crashes in glucose.
- Lean Proteins: Incorporating lean protein sources, such as poultry, fish, and legumes, into the DASH diet supports balanced blood sugar levels and contributes to insulin sensitivity.
- Healthy Fats: The inclusion of heart-healthy fats, like those found in nuts, seeds, and olive oil, helps slow down the digestion of carbohydrates and prevents sudden blood sugar spikes.
- Weight Management: Maintaining a healthy weight through the DASH diet can have a positive impact on diabetes management, as excess weight

is often associated with insulin resistance.

DASH Diet for Heart Health: Reducing Cholesterol and Cardiovascular Risks

Beyond its benefits for blood pressure management, the DASH diet plays a significant role in improving overall heart health and reducing cardiovascular risks.

- Cholesterol Reduction: The DASH diet's emphasis on lean proteins, low-fat dairy products, and healthy fats contributes to lower levels of LDL ("bad") cholesterol and higher levels of HDL ("good") cholesterol.
- Inflammation Reduction: The anti-inflammatory properties of the DASH diet, derived from its abundance of fruits, vegetables, and healthy fats, help reduce inflammation in the body—a key factor in cardiovascular disease.
- Blood Vessel Health: The combination of nutrients in the DASH diet, including potassium, magnesium, and antioxidants, supports blood vessel health and contributes to improved circulation.
- Weight Management: Maintaining a healthy weight through the DASH diet reduces the strain on the cardiovascular system and lowers the risk of heart disease.

In conclusion, the DASH diet offers a multifaceted approach to health that extends beyond blood pressure management. By incorporating nutrient-rich foods, controlling portion sizes, and making mindful dietary choices, individuals can harness the power of the DASH diet to promote weight management, control blood sugar levels, and reduce the risk of heart disease and other chronic conditions.

Practical Tips for Success
Grocery Shopping: Making DASH-Friendly Choices

Effective grocery shopping is a fundamental step in successfully adopting and maintaining the DASH diet. By making mindful choices at the store, you can ensure that your kitchen is stocked with nutrient-rich ingredients that align with the principles of the DASH diet.

- Plan Ahead: Before heading to the store, create a shopping list based on DASH-friendly recipes and meals you plan to prepare. Having a list helps you stay focused and avoid impulse purchases of unhealthy items.
- Focus on Fresh Produce: Allocate a significant portion of your shopping list to fruits and vegetables. Opt for a variety of colors and types to ensure a diverse nutrient intake.
- Choose Whole Grains: Stock up on whole grain options like brown rice, quinoa, whole wheat pasta, and whole grain bread. These provide a source of complex carbohydrates and dietary fiber.
- Lean Proteins: Select lean protein sources such as skinless poultry, fish, beans, lentils, and tofu. These options are lower in saturated fat and align with the DASH diet's protein recommendations.
- Low-Fat Dairy: Choose low-fat or fat-free dairy products like yogurt, milk, and cheese. Alternatively, consider dairy alternatives fortified with calcium and vitamin D.
- Minimize Processed Foods: Avoid heavily

processed and high-sodium foods, as they conflict with the DASH diet's focus on whole and minimally processed options.

- Read Labels: Pay attention to food labels to identify sodium content and select products with lower sodium levels.

Meal Prepping and Batch Cooking for Busy Lifestyles

Incorporating meal prepping and batch cooking into your routine can be a game-changer when following the DASH diet, especially for those with busy schedules. These strategies help you stay on track, save time, and ensure you have healthy meals readily available.

- Plan Your Menu: Choose DASH-compliant recipes for the week ahead. Plan meals that include a variety of food groups and nutrients.
- Prep Ingredients: Wash, chop, and portion fruits, vegetables, and proteins in advance. Store them in airtight containers for easy access.
- Cook in Batches: Prepare larger quantities of staple foods like whole grains, lean proteins, and vegetables. Store them separately and combine them to create balanced meals throughout the week.
- Portion Control: Use portioned containers to help you visualize appropriate serving sizes and prevent overeating.
- Freezing: Freeze individual portions of soups, stews, and other dishes for convenient meals on busy days.

Dining Out the DASH Way: Navigating Restaurant Menus

Maintaining the DASH diet while dining out requires a bit of preparation and awareness, but it's entirely possible to make health-conscious choices at restaurants.

- Preview the Menu: Check out the restaurant's menu online before going. Look for items that align with DASH principles, such as grilled lean proteins, salads, and vegetable-based dishes.
- Customize Your Order: Don't hesitate to ask for substitutions or modifications to make a dish more DASH-friendly. Request grilled options instead of fried, and ask for dressings and sauces on the side.
- Control Portions: Restaurant portions tend to be larger than what you might eat at home. Consider sharing a dish or asking for a to-go box to pack up half of your meal before you start eating.
- Sides and Add-Ons: Opt for vegetable sides, brown rice, or whole grain options instead of fries or refined grains.
- Beverage Choices: Choose water, unsweetened tea, or other low-calorie beverages instead of sugary drinks or high-calorie cocktails.

Overcoming Challenges: Staying Consistent with the DASH Diet

Adopting a new dietary pattern can come with its challenges, but with determination and the right strategies, you can stay consistent with the DASH diet.

- Educate Yourself: Continuously learn about the DASH diet, its benefits, and how it supports your health goals. Understanding the science behind the diet can motivate you to stick with it.

- Set Realistic Goals: Establish achievable goals that align with your lifestyle and preferences. Whether it's gradually reducing sodium intake or incorporating more vegetables, small changes add up over time.
- Mindful Eating: Practice mindful eating to become more attuned to hunger and fullness cues. This helps prevent overeating and encourages a healthier relationship with food.
- Stay Prepared: Keep DASH-friendly snacks on hand to avoid reaching for less nutritious options when hunger strikes unexpectedly.
- Seek Support: Enlist the support of friends, family, or a healthcare professional. Sharing your goals and progress with others can help keep you accountable.
- Celebrate Progress: Acknowledge your achievements and milestones along the way. Celebrate your successes, whether they're small dietary changes or larger health improvements.

Adapting to the DASH diet and integrating it into your daily life takes time and effort, but the rewards are well worth it. By making informed grocery choices, practicing meal prepping, navigating dining out, and addressing challenges with determination, you can successfully embrace the DASH diet and enjoy its myriad health benefits.

Lifestyle Integration and Long-Term Benefits
DASH Diet as a Lifestyle, Not a Fad

One of the key differentiators of the DASH diet is its focus on long-term health and sustainability, positioning it as a lifestyle choice rather than a temporary fad. Unlike quick-fix diets that promise rapid results, the DASH diet offers a holistic approach to nutrition that promotes overall well-being and prevents chronic diseases over time.

- Nutrient-Rich Eating: The DASH diet encourages a balanced intake of whole foods, providing essential nutrients that support various bodily functions and contribute to overall health.
- Sustainable Weight Management: By prioritizing portion control, balanced meals, and nutrient-dense foods, the DASH diet offers a realistic and effective approach to weight management that can be maintained over the long term.
- Disease Prevention: The DASH diet's emphasis on heart-healthy foods, blood pressure regulation, and blood sugar control reduces the risk of chronic conditions such as hypertension, diabetes, and cardiovascular diseases.
- Flexible and Adaptable: The DASH diet is adaptable to various dietary preferences and cultural backgrounds, making it a versatile choice for individuals seeking a healthy eating pattern.

Physical Activity and Exercise: Enhancing DASH Diet Results

Physical activity and exercise complement the DASH diet's principles, enhancing its benefits and promoting optimal health. Regular physical activity aligns with the DASH diet's goals of managing blood pressure, weight, and overall well-being.

- Cardiovascular Health: Both the DASH diet and exercise contribute to improved cardiovascular health, reducing the risk of heart disease and related complications.

- Weight Management: Combining the DASH diet with regular exercise supports weight loss, muscle maintenance, and metabolism, leading to more effective and sustainable results.
- Blood Sugar Regulation: Physical activity improves insulin sensitivity, helping individuals better manage blood sugar levels—especially relevant for those with diabetes or at risk of developing the condition.
- Stress Reduction: Exercise is a natural stress reliever, complementing the DASH diet's holistic approach to health by addressing both physical and mental well-being.

Stress Management and Sleep: Holistic Approaches to Health

Incorporating stress management techniques and prioritizing quality sleep aligns with the DASH diet's holistic approach to health. Addressing these aspects of well-being complements the diet's goals of blood pressure management and overall cardiovascular health.

- Stress Reduction: Chronic stress can contribute to high blood pressure and other health issues. Practices such as meditation, deep breathing, and mindfulness can help manage stress and promote relaxation.
- Healthy Sleep Habits: Prioritizing adequate sleep supports overall health and well-being, including blood pressure regulation, immune function, and cognitive performance.

- Mind-Body Connection: Integrating stress reduction and quality sleep into your routine enhances the DASH diet's effectiveness by addressing the interconnectedness of physical and mental health.

Celebrating Success: Tracking Progress and Staying Motivated

Tracking progress and celebrating successes are essential components of maintaining motivation and adherence to the DASH diet. Monitoring your journey helps you stay focused on your goals and recognize the positive changes you're making.

- Food Diary: Keeping a food diary allows you to track your meals, portion sizes, and nutrient intake. This practice promotes mindful eating and helps identify areas for improvement.
- Physical Activity Log: Documenting your exercise routine and physical activity achievements can boost motivation and provide a sense of accomplishment.
- Health Metrics: Regularly monitoring blood pressure, weight, and other relevant health metrics helps you track improvements and stay accountable to your health goals.
- Non-Scale Victories: Celebrate non-scale victories, such as increased energy levels, improved mood, better sleep, and enhanced overall well-being.
- Support System: Share your successes with friends, family, or a support group. Their encouragement and recognition can bolster your motivation and commitment to the DASH diet

and a healthier lifestyle.

Embracing the DASH diet as a holistic lifestyle choice, integrating physical activity and exercise, managing stress, prioritizing sleep, and celebrating your achievements contribute to a well-rounded and sustainable approach to health and well-being. By adopting these practices, you can maximize the benefits of the DASH diet and enjoy a vibrant and fulfilling life.

Frequently Asked Questions about the DASH Diet
Is the DASH Diet Suitable for Everyone?

The DASH diet is generally considered a healthy and balanced eating pattern that can benefit many individuals. However, it's important to note that individual dietary needs can vary based on factors such as medical conditions, lifestyle, preferences, and cultural considerations. Here are some points to consider when determining if the DASH diet is suitable for you:

- Medical Conditions: The DASH diet is particularly recommended for those with high blood pressure or at risk of developing hypertension. It can also be beneficial for individuals with diabetes, heart disease, and weight management goals.
- Dietary Preferences: The DASH diet is flexible and can be adapted to various dietary preferences, including vegetarian and vegan diets. However, some individuals may need to modify the diet to meet specific needs, such as dairy allergies or gluten intolerance.
- Cultural Considerations: The DASH diet's emphasis on whole foods, fruits, vegetables,

lean proteins, and whole grains can align well with many cultural cuisines. Modifications can be made to incorporate traditional foods while adhering to DASH principles.

Consultation with a Healthcare Professional: Before making significant dietary changes, especially if you have existing health conditions, it's advisable to consult with a healthcare professional or registered dietitian. They can provide personalized guidance and ensure that the DASH diet is appropriate for your individual situation.

Can I Follow the DASH Diet on a Budget?

Yes, it is possible to follow the DASH diet on a budget by making strategic food choices and planning your meals thoughtfully. Here are some tips to help you adopt the DASH diet without breaking the bank:

- Buy in Bulk: Purchase staple items like whole grains, legumes, and frozen fruits and vegetables in bulk. This can be cost-effective and reduce waste.
- Seasonal and Local Produce: Opt for seasonal and locally grown fruits and vegetables, as they tend to be more affordable and fresher.
- Plant-Based Proteins: Incorporate cost-effective plant-based protein sources like beans, lentils, tofu, and eggs.
- Sales and Coupons: Take advantage of sales, discounts, and coupons to save on items like whole grains, canned vegetables, and lean proteins.
- Meal Planning: Plan your meals in advance to avoid impulse purchases and minimize food

waste.

- Generic Brands: Consider purchasing store-brand or generic products, which are often more budget-friendly than name-brand options.

How Does the DASH Diet Compare to Other Popular Diets?

The DASH diet stands out among popular diets for its focus on overall health and its specific emphasis on reducing blood pressure. While other diets may prioritize weight loss or specific macronutrient ratios, the DASH diet takes a comprehensive approach to nutrition and well-being.

- Compared to Low-Carb Diets: Low-carb diets may limit carbohydrate intake, which can affect energy levels and may not be suitable for everyone. The DASH diet includes a balance of carbohydrates, protein, and healthy fats, making it more sustainable for the long term.
- Compared to Mediterranean Diet: The DASH diet shares similarities with the Mediterranean diet, including an emphasis on fruits, vegetables, whole grains, and lean proteins. However, the DASH diet places a stronger focus on reducing sodium intake to manage blood pressure.
- Compared to Keto Diet: The ketogenic (keto) diet is very low in carbohydrates and high in fat, which may not align with the balanced approach of the DASH diet. The DASH diet promotes a variety of nutrient-rich foods and encourages whole grains, which provide essential nutrients and dietary fiber.

Addressing Common Misconceptions about the DASH Diet

There are a few misconceptions about the DASH diet that are worth addressing to provide a clear understanding of its principles and benefits:

- Not Just for Hypertension: While the DASH diet is renowned for its effectiveness in managing blood pressure, its nutrient-rich and balanced approach to eating can benefit individuals without hypertension as well.
- Not a Quick Fix: The DASH diet is not a quick-fix solution for weight loss or health improvement. It's a long-term lifestyle approach that emphasizes sustainable changes and overall well-being.
- Flexibility and Variety: Some may assume that the DASH diet is restrictive, but it offers flexibility and encourages a wide variety of foods. It can be adapted to different dietary preferences and cultural backgrounds.
- Holistic Health: The DASH diet is more than just a dietary plan; it incorporates factors such as stress management, physical activity, and sleep, acknowledging the interconnectedness of overall health.

In conclusion, understanding the suitability of the DASH diet for different individuals, its feasibility on a budget, its unique attributes compared to other diets, and addressing common misconceptions can provide a comprehensive perspective on the diet's benefits and practicality. Always consult with a healthcare professional or registered dietitian before making significant dietary changes to ensure they align with your specific health goals and needs.

Your Journey to Better Health with the DASH Diet

Setting Personal Goals: Tailoring DASH to Your Needs

Setting personal goals is a crucial step in tailoring the DASH diet to your individual needs and ensuring its effectiveness in achieving your desired outcomes. By identifying specific objectives, you can customize your approach and stay motivated on your journey to better health.

- Identify Your Priorities: Determine what aspects of your health you want to focus on. Whether it's blood pressure management, weight loss, better blood sugar control, or overall well-being, clarifying your priorities helps you set targeted goals.
- Be Realistic: Set achievable and realistic goals that align with your current lifestyle and circumstances. Avoid setting overly ambitious targets that might lead to frustration or burnout.
- Break It Down: Divide your goals into smaller, manageable steps. This approach makes your objectives more attainable and allows you to track progress along the way.
- Make It Measurable: Frame your goals in a way that can be measured and tracked. For instance, aim to increase your daily intake of vegetables or reduce your sodium intake to a specific amount.

Monitoring Progress: Tracking Health Metrics and Adjusting Strategies

Monitoring your progress is essential to gauge the effectiveness of your efforts and make informed adjustments to your DASH diet and lifestyle strategies. Regularly tracking health metrics and other indicators helps you stay on course and make necessary modifications.

- Health Metrics: Keep tabs on key health indicators, such as blood pressure, weight, cholesterol levels, and blood sugar. Regular check-ins with your healthcare provider can provide valuable insights into your progress.
- Food Journal: Maintain a food journal to record your meals, snacks, and portion sizes. This practice enhances mindfulness and helps identify patterns that may impact your goals.
- Physical Activity Log: Keep track of your exercise routine and activity levels. Monitoring your physical activity helps you ensure that you're meeting your fitness goals.
- Regular Assessments: Set aside specific times, such as monthly or quarterly, to assess your progress and adjust your strategies if needed. If you're not seeing the desired results, consider consulting with a healthcare professional or registered dietitian for guidance.

Sustaining Long-Term Success: Making DASH a Lifelong Habit

Making the DASH diet a lifelong habit is key to sustaining long-term success and reaping its ongoing health benefits. Incorporate the following strategies to integrate the DASH principles into your daily routine and make it a sustainable way of life:

- Consistency: Consistency is key to long-term success. Aim to consistently follow DASH principles while allowing occasional flexibility to accommodate special occasions or personal preferences.
- Gradual Changes: Gradually integrate DASH-friendly habits into your routine. Making small, incremental changes over time is more sustainable than attempting drastic shifts all at once.
- Mindful Eating: Embrace mindful eating practices by paying attention to hunger and fullness cues, savoring each bite, and avoiding distractions during meals.
- Meal Planning: Continue to plan your meals and snacks ahead of time. Meal prepping and having nutritious options readily available reduce the likelihood of making less healthy choices.
- Support System: Enlist the support of friends, family, or a community with similar goals. Sharing your journey and challenges with others can provide motivation, accountability, and a sense of camaraderie.
- Flexibility: Be adaptable and open to adjustments as your circumstances change. Life events, travel, and other factors may require modifications to your routine while still staying true to DASH principles.

Incorporating personal goals, monitoring progress, and sustaining the DASH diet as a lifelong habit empower you to make lasting improvements to your health and well-being. By taking a holistic and individualized approach, you can successfully integrate the principles of the DASH diet into your lifestyle and enjoy the benefits for years to come.

CHAPTER THREE
Greek Yogurt Parfait with Mixed Berries and a Sprinkle of Nuts
Description of the Meal:

Indulge in a delightful Greek yogurt parfait that's bursting with flavors and textures. This vibrant creation combines creamy Greek yogurt with a medley of mixed berries, and a generous sprinkle of assorted nuts for a satisfying crunch.

Ingredients:

- 1 cup of Greek yogurt
- ½ cup of mixed berries (strawberries, blueberries, raspberries)
- 2 tablespoons of chopped nuts (almonds, walnuts, pistachios)
- A drizzle of honey for sweetness (optional)

Instructions:

- Start by layering a spoonful of Greek yogurt at the bottom of a glass or bowl.
- Add a handful of mixed berries on top of the yogurt layer.

- Repeat the layering process with yogurt and berries until the container is almost full.
- Sprinkle the chopped nuts over the final layer for a delightful crunch.
- Optionally, drizzle honey over the top for added sweetness.
- Enjoy this parfait with a spoon, savoring the contrast of creamy yogurt, juicy berries, and nutty textures.

Nutritional Information:

Calories: 250

Protein: 15g

Carbohydrates: 30g

Fat: 10g

Fiber: 5g

Oatmeal Topped with Sliced Bananas, Chopped Walnuts, and a Drizzle of Honey

Description of the Meal:

Warm up your morning with a comforting bowl of oatmeal, adorned with the natural sweetness of sliced bananas, the crunch of chopped walnuts, and a delicate drizzle of golden honey.

Ingredients:

- ½ cup of rolled oats
- 1 cup of water or milk (dairy or plant-based)
- 1 ripe banana, sliced
- 2 tablespoons of chopped walnuts
- 1 teaspoon of honey

Instructions:

- In a saucepan, bring the water or milk to a gentle boil.
- Add the rolled oats and stir, then reduce the heat to a simmer.
- Cook the oats for about 5 minutes or until they reach your desired consistency.
- Once cooked, transfer the oatmeal to a bowl.
- Arrange the sliced banana on top of the oatmeal.
- Sprinkle the chopped walnuts over the banana slices.
- Finish by drizzling a teaspoon of honey over the toppings.
- Mix everything together before indulging in the delightful combination of textures and flavors.

Nutritional Information:

Calories: 350

Protein: 8g

Carbohydrates: 55g

Fat: 12g

Fiber: 7g

Veggie Omelette with Spinach, Tomatoes, and Bell Peppers

Description of the Meal:

Dive into a colorful and nutritious veggie omelette that's bursting with vibrant flavors. This wholesome creation features a fluffy egg base folded around sautéed spinach, juicy tomatoes, and crisp bell peppers.

Ingredients:

- 3 eggs
- ¼ cup of fresh spinach, chopped
- ¼ cup of tomatoes, diced
- ¼ cup of bell peppers, diced
- Salt and pepper to taste
- 1 teaspoon of olive oil

Instructions:

- Crack the eggs into a bowl and whisk them until well combined.
- Heat olive oil in a non-stick skillet over medium heat.
- Sauté the diced tomatoes and bell peppers until slightly softened.
- Add the chopped spinach to the skillet and cook until wilted.
- Pour the whisked eggs over the cooked vegetables in the skillet.
- Cook the omelette until the edges set, then gently fold it in half.
- Continue cooking for another minute or until the eggs are fully cooked.
- Season with salt and pepper to taste.
- Slide the omelette onto a plate and admire the burst of colors before savoring every bite.

Nutritional Information:

Calories: 220

Protein: 15g

Carbohydrates: 8g

Fat: 15g

Fiber: 2g

Whole-Grain Toast with Avocado Spread and Poached Eggs

Description of the Meal:

Elevate your breakfast with a satisfying ensemble of whole-grain toast topped with creamy avocado spread and perfectly poached eggs. This combination offers a delightful mix of textures and rich flavors.

Ingredients:

- 2 slices of whole-grain bread, toasted
- 1 ripe avocado
- Juice of half a lemon
- Salt and pepper to taste
- 2 large eggs

Instructions:

- Cut the avocado in half, remove the pit, and scoop the flesh into a bowl.
- Mash the avocado with a fork and mix in the lemon juice, salt, and pepper.
- Poach the eggs using your preferred method until the whites are set but the yolks remain runny.
- Spread the avocado mixture evenly onto the toasted whole-grain bread slices.
- Gently place a poached egg on top of each toast slice.
- Sprinkle a pinch of salt and pepper over the eggs.
- Break the poached eggs open, allowing the luscious yolk to create a creamy contrast with the avocado spread.
- Enjoy this open-faced sandwich with a fork and knife, relishing the harmonious blend of textures

and flavors.

Nutritional Information:

Calories: 350

Protein: 15g

Carbohydrates: 30g

Fat: 20g

Fiber: 10g

Cottage Cheese with Sliced Peaches and a Side of Whole-Grain Toast

Description of the Meal:

Savor the simplicity of this wholesome meal featuring cottage cheese, luscious sliced peaches, and a side of hearty whole-grain toast. The combination of creamy, sweet, and nutty flavors will leave you feeling satisfied and nourished.

Ingredients:

- 1 cup of cottage cheese
- 1 ripe peach, sliced
- 2 slices of whole-grain bread, toasted

Instructions:

- Start by placing a generous scoop of cottage cheese in a bowl.
- Arrange the sliced peaches on one side of the bowl.
- Toast the whole-grain bread slices until they're golden and crispy.
- Serve the toast on the side, providing a hearty crunch to complement the creamy cottage cheese and juicy peaches.
- Alternate between bites of cottage cheese, peach

slices, and bites of toast, relishing the delightful contrast of flavors and textures.

Nutritional Information:

Calories: 300

Protein: 20g

Carbohydrates: 35g

Fat: 8g

Fiber: 5g

Tuna Salad with Mixed Greens, Cherry Tomatoes, and a Lemon-Olive Oil Dressing

Description of the Meal:

Indulge in a refreshing tuna salad, featuring a medley of mixed greens, juicy cherry tomatoes, and a zesty lemon-olive oil dressing. This salad brings together the richness of tuna, the crispness of greens, and the vibrant flavors of a citrus-infused dressing.

Ingredients:

- 4 oz canned tuna, drained
- 2 cups mixed greens (romaine, iceberg, spring mix)
- ½ cup cherry tomatoes, halved
- 2 tablespoons olive oil
- Juice of 1 lemon
- Salt and pepper to taste

Instructions:

- In a bowl, combine the mixed greens and cherry tomato halves.
- Flake the canned tuna and scatter it over the

- greens.
- In a separate bowl, whisk together the olive oil, lemon juice, salt, and pepper to create the dressing.
- Drizzle the lemon-olive oil dressing over the salad.
- Toss gently to coat the ingredients with the dressing and distribute the flavors.
- Enjoy this refreshing salad, savoring each bite that combines the delicate notes of tuna with the vibrant greens and zesty dressing.

Nutritional Information:

Calories: 300

Protein: 25g

Carbohydrates: 10g

Fat: 18g

Fiber: 4g

Grilled Chicken Salad with Mixed Greens, Cucumbers, Carrots, and Balsamic Vinaigrette

Description of the Meal:

Experience a burst of freshness with this grilled chicken salad, featuring a colorful array of mixed greens, crisp cucumbers, and vibrant carrots. Topped with tender grilled chicken and drizzled with tangy balsamic vinaigrette, this salad is a harmonious symphony of flavors.

Ingredients:

- 4 oz grilled chicken breast, sliced
- 2 cups mixed greens (lettuce, arugula, spinach)
- ½ cucumber, sliced
- 1 carrot, julienned

- 2 tablespoons balsamic vinaigrette dressing

Instructions:

- Arrange the mixed greens on a serving plate.
- Scatter cucumber slices and julienned carrots over the greens.
- Place the sliced grilled chicken on top of the salad.
- Drizzle the balsamic vinaigrette dressing over the entire salad.
- Toss gently to combine all the ingredients and coat them with the dressing.
- Relish each bite, savoring the crispness of the vegetables, the tenderness of the chicken, and the tangy notes of the vinaigrette.

Nutritional Information:

Calories: 350

Protein: 30g

Carbohydrates: 15g

Fat: 18g

Fiber: 4g

Quinoa and Black Bean Bowl with Roasted Vegetables and a Squeeze of Lime

Description of the Meal:

Delight in a hearty and wholesome quinoa and black bean bowl, adorned with roasted vegetables and a zesty squeeze of lime. This bowl combines the nutty goodness of quinoa, the earthy flavor of black beans, and the vibrant colors of assorted roasted vegetables.

Ingredients:

- 1 cup cooked quinoa
- ½ cup black beans, drained and rinsed
- 1 cup roasted vegetables (bell peppers, zucchini, red onion)
- Juice of 1 lime
- Salt and pepper to taste

Instructions:

- In a bowl, layer the cooked quinoa as the base.
- Spoon the black beans over the quinoa.
- Arrange the roasted vegetables on top of the beans.
- Squeeze the lime juice over the entire bowl.
- Season with salt and pepper to taste.
- Gently mix the ingredients together, allowing the flavors to meld.
- Dive into this nourishing bowl, relishing the interplay of textures and the vibrant medley of flavors.

Nutritional Information:

Calories: 400

Protein: 15g

Carbohydrates: 65g

Fat: 8g

Fiber: 12g

Turkey and Avocado Wrap with Whole-Grain Tortilla and a Side of Carrot Sticks
Description of the Meal:

Indulge in a delightful turkey and avocado wrap, nestled within a whole-grain tortilla and accompanied by a refreshing side of carrot sticks. This wrap offers a satisfying balance of lean turkey, creamy avocado, and the crunch of fresh vegetables.

Ingredients:

- 4 oz turkey breast slices
- ½ avocado, sliced
- 1 whole-grain tortilla
- 1 carrot, cut into sticks

Instructions:

- Lay the whole-grain tortilla flat on a clean surface.
- Arrange the turkey slices and avocado slices down the center of the tortilla.
- Roll the tortilla tightly around the fillings to form a wrap.
- Slice the wrap diagonally for easier handling.
- Serve the wrap alongside a handful of carrot sticks.
- Take a bite of the wrap followed by a satisfying crunch of carrot sticks, savoring the combination of textures and flavors.

Nutritional Information:

Calories: 350

Protein: 25g

Carbohydrates: 30g

Fat: 15g

Fiber: 7g

Lentil Soup with a Side of Whole-Grain Roll and a Mixed Green Salad

Description of the Meal:

Warm your soul with a comforting bowl of lentil soup, complemented by a wholesome whole-grain roll and a refreshing mixed green salad. This meal combines the heartiness of lentils, the warmth of soup, and the crispness of fresh greens.

Ingredients:

- 1 cup lentil soup (homemade or store-bought)
- 1 whole-grain roll
- Mixed greens (lettuce, baby spinach, arugula)
- Your favorite salad toppings (cherry tomatoes, cucumber, red onion)

Instructions:

- Heat the lentil soup in a pot until it's steaming hot.
- Warm the whole-grain roll in the oven or toaster.
- In a bowl, assemble a mix of your preferred greens.
- Add your choice of salad toppings for extra crunch and flavor.
- Serve the lentil soup in a bowl, accompanied by the whole-grain roll and the mixed green salad.
- Dip the roll into the soup and take alternating bites of soup and salad, enjoying the nourishing combination of flavors and textures.

Nutritional Information:

Calories: 450

Protein: 20g

Carbohydrates: 80g

Fat: 5g

Fiber: 15g

Baked Salmon with Steamed Broccoli and Quinoa

Description of the Meal:

Indulge in a wholesome feast with this baked salmon dish, accompanied by tender steamed broccoli and fluffy quinoa. This combination offers a symphony of flavors, textures, and nourishing goodness.

Ingredients:

- 6 oz salmon fillet
- 1 cup steamed broccoli florets
- ½ cup cooked quinoa
- Lemon slices for garnish
- Fresh dill or parsley for garnish

Instructions:

- Preheat the oven to 375°F (190°C).
- Place the salmon fillet on a baking sheet lined with parchment paper.
- Season the salmon with salt, pepper, and your choice of herbs.
- Bake the salmon in the preheated oven for 15-20 minutes or until cooked to your desired level of doneness.
- While the salmon is baking, steam the broccoli until tender-crisp.
- Prepare the quinoa according to package instructions.
- Once everything is ready, arrange the baked salmon on a plate.
- Serve with a side of steamed broccoli and a scoop of cooked quinoa.

- Garnish with lemon slices and fresh dill or parsley.
- Delight in the succulent salmon, the vibrant broccoli, and the nutty quinoa, relishing the harmonious combination.

Nutritional Information:

Calories: 400

Protein: 35g

Carbohydrates: 30g

Fat: 15g

Fiber: 5g

Grilled Vegetable Stir-Fry with Tofu and Brown Rice

Description of the Meal:

Embark on a culinary adventure with this vibrant grilled vegetable stir-fry, featuring marinated tofu and wholesome brown rice. Immerse yourself in the delightful blend of smoky grilled flavors and the heartiness of plant-based protein.

Ingredients:

- 6 oz firm tofu, cubed
- Assorted grilled vegetables (bell peppers, zucchini, eggplant, onion)
- 1 cup cooked brown rice
- Stir-fry sauce (soy sauce, ginger, garlic, sesame oil)
- Sesame seeds for garnish

Instructions:

- Marinate the tofu cubes in your choice of stir-fry sauce for at least 15 minutes.

- Grill the marinated tofu until lightly browned and cooked through.
- In a separate pan, stir-fry the grilled vegetables until tender.
- Reheat the cooked brown rice.
- Combine the grilled vegetables, tofu, and brown rice in a large bowl.
- Drizzle with additional stir-fry sauce and toss to coat.
- Serve the grilled vegetable stir-fry, garnished with sesame seeds.
- Dive into this explosion of flavors, embracing the smokiness of the grilled vegetables and the savory notes of the tofu.

Nutritional Information:

Calories: 420

Protein: 20g

Carbohydrates: 60g

Fat: 12g

Fiber: 8g

Lemon Herb Grilled Chicken with Roasted Sweet Potatoes and Asparagus

Description of the Meal:

Experience a symphony of flavors with this lemon herb grilled chicken, accompanied by roasted sweet potatoes and tender asparagus. This dish marries the succulence of grilled chicken with the sweetness of roasted root vegetables.

Ingredients:

- 6 oz chicken breast
- 1 medium sweet potato, cubed
- 1 bunch of asparagus, trimmed
- Lemon slices for garnish
- Fresh herbs (thyme, rosemary, or parsley) for garnish

Instructions:

- Marinate the chicken breast in a lemon herb marinade for about 30 minutes.
- Preheat the oven to 400°F (200°C).
- Toss the cubed sweet potatoes with a drizzle of olive oil and your choice of herbs.
- Roast the sweet potatoes in the preheated oven for 20-25 minutes, until golden and tender.
- Grill the marinated chicken breast until cooked through and no longer pink in the center.
- While grilling the chicken, lightly steam the asparagus until crisp-tender.
- Arrange the grilled chicken on a plate, surrounded by roasted sweet potatoes and steamed asparagus.
- Garnish with lemon slices and fresh herbs.
- Revel in the flavorful combination of the succulent chicken, the caramelized sweet potatoes, and the vibrant asparagus.

Nutritional Information:

Calories: 450

Protein: 40g

Carbohydrates: 35g

Fat: 15g

Fiber: 8g

Spaghetti Squash with Marinara Sauce and a Side of Mixed Greens

Description of the Meal:

Delight in a unique twist on traditional pasta with this spaghetti squash dish, accompanied by a rich marinara sauce and a refreshing side of mixed greens. This meal offers a lighter alternative while delivering robust Italian flavors.

Ingredients:

- 1 small spaghetti squash
- 1 cup marinara sauce (homemade or store-bought)
- Mixed greens (lettuce, arugula, spinach)
- Balsamic vinaigrette for dressing

Instructions:

- Preheat the oven to 375°F (190°C).
- Cut the spaghetti squash in half lengthwise and scoop out the seeds.
- Place the spaghetti squash halves, cut side down, on a baking sheet.
- Roast in the preheated oven for 30-40 minutes or until the strands can be easily scraped with a fork.
- Scrape the flesh of the spaghetti squash with a fork to create "spaghetti" strands.
- Heat the marinara sauce in a saucepan.
- Serve the spaghetti squash with a ladle of marinara sauce on top.
- Accompany the dish with a side of mixed greens.
- Drizzle the mixed greens with balsamic vinaigrette for a refreshing contrast.

- Enjoy this guilt-free, low-carb alternative that captures the essence of traditional Italian comfort food.

Nutritional Information:

Calories: 250

Protein: 6g

Carbohydrates: 40g

Fat: 8g

Fiber: 8g

Black Bean and Sweet Potato Enchiladas with a Side of Sautéed Spinach

Description of the Meal:

Savor the rich flavors of black bean and sweet potato enchiladas, complemented by a side of sautéed spinach. This dish embraces the warmth of Mexican cuisine and the nourishing goodness of wholesome ingredients.

Ingredients:

- 1 cup black beans, cooked and mashed
- 1 medium sweet potato, roasted and mashed
- 6 small corn tortillas
- Enchilada sauce (red or green)
- 1 cup fresh spinach leaves
- Lime wedges for garnish

Instructions:

- Preheat the oven to 375°F (190°C).
- In a bowl, combine the mashed black beans and roasted sweet potato.
- Soften the corn tortillas by heating them briefly in

a dry skillet.

- Place a spoonful of the black bean and sweet potato mixture in the center of each tortilla and roll them up.
- Place the rolled enchiladas in a baking dish and cover with enchilada sauce.
- Bake in the preheated oven for 20-25 minutes or until heated through.
- While the enchiladas are baking, sauté the spinach in a pan until wilted.
- Serve the enchiladas with a side of sautéed spinach and lime wedges.
- Enjoy the delectable combination of sweet and savory flavors, as well as the vibrant colors of this Mexican-inspired dish.

Nutritional Information:

Calories: 400

Protein: 10g

Carbohydrates: 70g

Fat: 8g

Fiber: 12g

Hummus with Baby Carrots, Celery, and Whole-Grain Crackers

Description of the Snack:

Dive into a wholesome and satisfying snack featuring creamy hummus, crisp baby carrots, crunchy celery, and whole-grain crackers. This combination offers a delightful balance of textures and flavors that will keep you energized and satisfied.

Ingredients:

½ cup hummus

- Baby carrots
- Celery sticks
- Whole-grain crackers

Instructions:

- Arrange the hummus in a bowl.
- Surround the hummus with baby carrots and celery sticks for dipping.
- Place whole-grain crackers alongside the vegetables.
- Dip the carrots, celery, and crackers into the hummus, savoring the contrast of creamy and crunchy textures.

Nutritional Information:

Calories: 250

Protein: 8g

Carbohydrates: 30g

Fat: 12g

Fiber: 8g

Apple Slices with Almond Butter
Description of the Snack:

Indulge in a delightful snack featuring crisp apple slices paired with velvety almond butter. This combination offers the natural sweetness of apples and the rich, nutty flavor of almond butter.

Ingredients:

- Apple, sliced
- Almond butter

Instructions:

- Slice the apple into thin wedges or rounds.
- Dip each apple slice into a dollop of almond butter.
- Relish the harmonious blend of flavors as you enjoy the satisfying crunch of the apple and the creamy almond butter.

Nutritional Information:

Calories: 200

Protein: 4g

Carbohydrates: 25g

Fat: 10g

Fiber: 6g

Mixed Nuts and Dried Fruit Trail Mix
Description of the Snack:

Experience a burst of energy with this trail mix featuring a medley of mixed nuts and dried fruits. This satisfying and nutrient-dense snack is perfect for on-the-go moments.

Ingredients:

- Assorted mixed nuts (almonds, walnuts, cashews)
- Dried fruits (raisins, cranberries, apricots)

Instructions:

- Combine a variety of mixed nuts in a bowl.
- Add a handful of dried fruits to the mix.
- Toss the nuts and dried fruits together to create a

flavorful and nourishing trail mix.

- Portion out the trail mix into small bags for convenient snacking throughout the day.

Nutritional Information:

Calories: 300

Protein: 8g

Carbohydrates: 20g

Fat: 22g

Fiber: 4g

Cottage Cheese with Pineapple Chunks
Description of the Snack:

Enjoy a refreshing and protein-packed snack with creamy cottage cheese and juicy pineapple chunks. This pairing brings together the creaminess of cottage cheese with the tropical sweetness of pineapple.

Ingredients:

- ½ cup cottage cheese
- Fresh pineapple chunks

Instructions:

- Spoon the cottage cheese into a bowl.
- Top the cottage cheese with a generous serving of fresh pineapple chunks.
- Dive into the creamy and sweet combination of cottage cheese and pineapple.

Nutritional Information:

Calories: 150

Protein: 15g

Carbohydrates: 20g

Fat: 2g

Fiber: 2g

Greek Yogurt with a Drizzle of Honey and a Handful of Granola

Description of the Snack:

Delight in the creamy goodness of Greek yogurt topped with a drizzle of honey and a handful of crunchy granola. This snack offers a delightful contrast of textures and a harmonious blend of flavors.

Ingredients:

- 1 cup Greek yogurt
- Honey for drizzling
- Handful of granola

Instructions:

- Spoon the Greek yogurt into a bowl.
- Drizzle honey over the yogurt for a touch of sweetness.
- Sprinkle a handful of granola on top for a satisfying crunch.
- Mix the ingredients together before enjoying each spoonful of creamy yogurt, honey, and granola.

Nutritional Information:

Calories: 300

Protein: 15g

Carbohydrates: 40g

Fat: 10g

Fiber: 5g

CONCLUSION

In a world where diets and health trends come and go, the Dietary Approaches to Stop Hypertension (DASH) diet stands as a beacon of sensible, science-backed nutrition. With a focus on overall well-being and the prevention of chronic diseases, the DASH diet offers a holistic approach to health that extends beyond mere weight loss. As we conclude our exploration of this dietary approach, let's reflect on the key takeaways and the profound impact the DASH diet can have on your life.

- A Blueprint for Health: The DASH diet provides a comprehensive blueprint for optimal health by emphasizing nutrient-rich foods, balanced meals, and a mindful approach to eating. It's not a quick-fix solution but a sustainable lifestyle that nourishes your body and supports your long-term well-being.
- Blood Pressure Management: At its core, the DASH diet is a potent tool for managing blood pressure. Through its careful selection of foods low in sodium and rich in potassium, calcium, and magnesium, the diet helps maintain healthy blood vessels and supports cardiovascular health.
- Beyond Blood Pressure: Yet, the DASH diet's benefits extend far beyond blood pressure management. It promotes weight loss and weight maintenance, making it an effective tool for

those seeking a healthier body composition. By regulating blood sugar levels and improving insulin sensitivity, it aids in diabetes prevention and management. Moreover, its emphasis on whole foods and antioxidants supports a strong immune system, reducing the risk of illness.

- Flexibility and Adaptability: The DASH diet's flexibility is a cornerstone of its success. Whether you're a meat-eater or a vegetarian, a busy professional or a stay-at-home parent, the DASH diet can be tailored to suit your preferences and lifestyle. With its emphasis on portion control, nutrient-dense foods, and mindful eating, it encourages a sustainable relationship with food that can be enjoyed for years to come.
- A Holistic Approach: The DASH diet is not just about what you eat—it's about how you live. It encourages regular physical activity, stress management, and quality sleep as integral components of a healthy lifestyle. By addressing these aspects, the DASH diet recognizes that true health is a holistic endeavor that encompasses both body and mind.

Your Journey to Embracing Health: As you embark on your journey to embrace health with the DASH diet, remember that progress is a series of small steps, each one contributing to a bigger picture of well-being. Whether you're aiming to lower your blood pressure, achieve a healthier weight, or simply lead a more vibrant life, the DASH diet offers a roadmap for success.

Celebrate every achievement, no matter how small. Whether it's choosing a nutrient-packed snack over a sugary indulgence or consistently incorporating more vegetables into your meals, these seemingly minor victories are building blocks that shape a healthier you.

In a world where health trends come and go, the DASH diet remains a steadfast beacon of evidence-based wisdom. Its principles transcend fads and offer a timeless path to lasting health and vitality. So, as you embrace the DASH diet and its principles, you are embarking on a transformative journey—one that will not only enhance your physical well-being but also empower you to lead a life brimming with energy, resilience, and joy. Here's to your health, to embracing the DASH diet, and to the vibrant future that lies ahead.